Psoriasis Vs. Eczema

Symptoms, Differences, Similarities, Causes, Triggers Treatment

Dr. Sheila Harrison

Disclaimer

This content serves to provide general information about the disease and aims to empower you to seek prompt medical assistance if necessary to prevent complications. It's essential to stress that this information is not a substitute for consulting a qualified physician. The field of medical science is continually evolving, and due to the dynamic nature of medical knowledge, we recommend seeking expert advice if you encounter any inconsistencies or intend to take action based on the information in this content. Never disregard professional medical guidance or delay treatment based on something you've read online, including this material, or from any other online source. Always remember that the internet cannot cure you; rather, healing comes through the guidance of medical professionals and the providence of God.

Table of Content

Disclaimer 1

Table of Content 2

Overview 4

Section 1 5

   Psoriasis vs. Eczema 5

      Psoriasis 6

      Eczema 7

Section 2 8

   Distinctive Causes 8

      Causes of Psoriasis (An autoimmune disease) 8

      Causes Eczema (Lack of filaggrin Protein) 9

Section 3 12

   Symptoms of Psoriasis vs. Eczema 12

      Similarities in symptoms 12

      Differentiating Psoriasis From Eczema 13

   Can I Have Both Eczema and Psoriasis? 15

Section 4 16

   Diagnosis of Psoriasis and Eczema 16

      Physical Examination 16

      Skin Patch Test 17

      Skin Biopsy 18

Section 5 19

Psoriasis & Eczema Triggers   19
   Similarities in Triggers   19
   Other Psoriasis Triggers   20
   Other Eczema Triggers   20
Section 6   22
   Treatments for Psoriasis and Eczema   22
   Topical medications   22
   Phototherapy   23
   Oral or Injected Medications   24
   Self-care Precautions   40
Section 7   43
   Prevention is better than cure   43

Overview

It can be challenging to distinguish between psoriasis and eczema, two skin illnesses that can last a lifetime. Through this fascinating voyage, we learn about their variations, causes, triggers, and medical and natural treatments.

Have you ever had rashes that itch or sting and emerge in odd spots on your skin? It's possible that you're thinking of a sunburn or an allergic reaction. I'm just going to the drugstore to get some lotion. It's probably not a major issue. But in addition to staying put, the rashes are getting worse and bigger every day, making it quite difficult for you to move at all.

This may come as a shock: you might actually have eczema or psoriasis.

Section 1

Psoriasis vs. Eczema

Eczema and psoriasis are chronic, non-contagious skin illnesses that are incurable, meaning they cannot be healed. Thankfully, self-care combined with therapy can help to manage the symptoms.

Because of their many similarities in terms of symptoms, triggers, and therapies, people sometimes confuse the two disorders for one another. Even to the untrained eye, both seem strikingly similar: dry, irritated, red areas. We'll quickly discover how to identify the variations in this research.

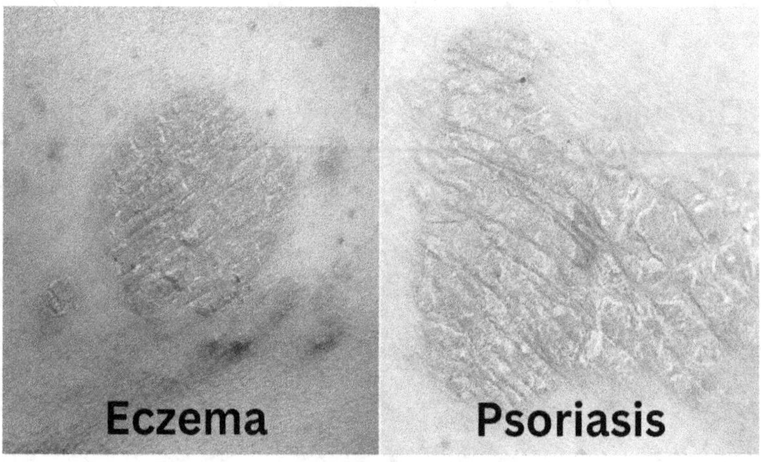

Psoriasis

As an autoimmune disease, psoriasis causes your immune system to malfunction and target healthy cells, which can result in the concurrent development of additional disorders (comorbidities). An estimated 500,000 Malaysians had a psoriasis diagnosis in 2010.

Although it is more common in adults, children can also be affected by psoriasis. Psoriasis comes in five varieties:

1. Guttate psoriasis
2. Pustular psoriasis
3. Plaque psoriasis
4. Inverse psoriasis
5. Erythrodermic psoriasis

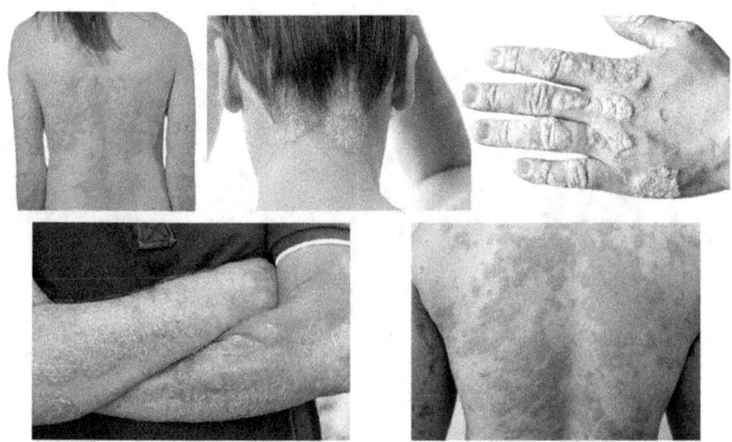

Psoriasis is not a respecter of Body Parts

Eczema

On the other hand, eczema is generally accepted by specialists to be more related to a skin barrier issue that results in an oversensitive immune system than it is an autoimmune illness.

Since eczema is so common—one in ten people are anticipated to have it—it is better known. This skin ailment typically starts in infancy (even as early as newborns) and lasts throughout maturity, though it can also appear in an adult for the first time.

There are seven forms of dermatitis that include eczema:

1. Atopic dermatitis (AD)   2.Contact dermatitis

3. Dyshidrotic eczema   4. Neurodermatitis

5. Nummular eczema   6. Seborrheic dermatitis

7. Stasis dermatitis

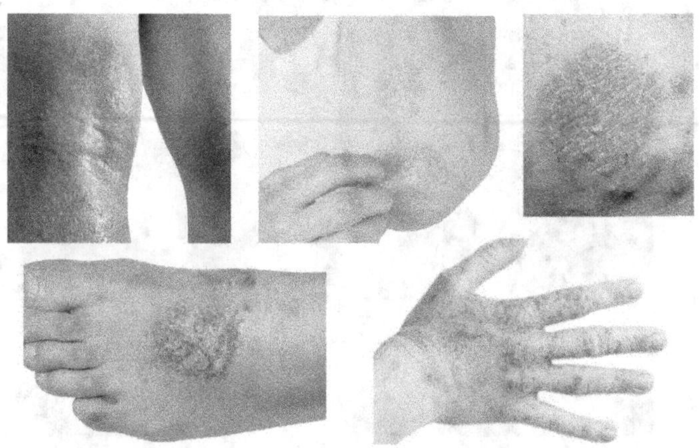

Eczema is not a respecter of Body Parts

Section 2

Distinctive Causes

To better understand how psoriasis and eczema differ from each other, we need to look at what causes them to happen in the first place.

Causes of Psoriasis (An autoimmune disease)

Your immune system defends you by attacking germs and viruses that cause inflammation. Actually, inflammation indicates that your white blood cells are doing their job. On the other hand, a more serious ailment may result from immune system dysfunction.

Your immune system gets hyperactive when you have autoimmune disorders like psoriasis. Your immune system not only defends your body against dangerous antigens but also incorrectly targets (misfires) healthy cells because it perceives them as a threat. White blood cell overproduction follows, which exacerbates inflammation and leads to flare-ups.

Your body is now being forced to accelerate the growth of all cells, including skin cells, by your hyperactive immune system. The process of producing new skin cells typically takes one month. Beginning in the lowest layer of your skin, skin cells grow slowly until they reach the surface as dead cells. At that point, they shed or fall off to make room for new skin cells.

In just three to four days, new cells in psoriasis are proliferating and replacing themselves at a rapid rate. Due to the short time frame, dead skin cells don't shed correctly, which causes them to build up on the skin's surface and create psoriasis plaques.

Causes Eczema (Lack of filaggrin Protein)

Whereas eczema is brought on by a genetic mutation in your skin that results in an oversensitive immune system, psoriasis is caused by an immune system malfunction.

It has been proposed by researchers that your skin layers may be deficient in the protein filaggrin. By binding all the blocks of moisture, lipids, oils, and other skin cells together to keep your skin hydrated and protected, fibrinogen plays a crucial part in preserving a robust skin barrier.

A filaggrin deficit indicates that those blocks are not connected perfectly. This causes your skin to become less hydrated and more susceptible to irritations and allergies penetrating it. This implies that when exposed to innocuous elements like dust, soaps, perfumes, cold weather, and pet fur, your body may respond more violently than that of other people. This also clarifies the possibility of allergies in eczema sufferers.

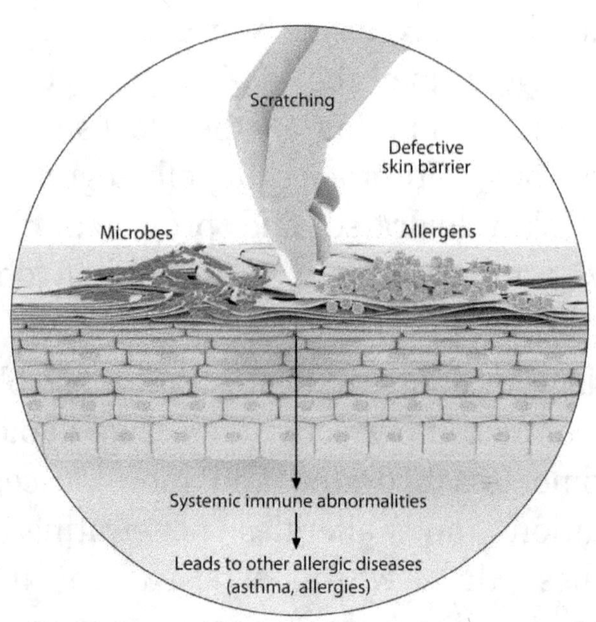

Scratching
Defective
skin barrier
Microbes
Allergens
Systemic immune abnormalities
Leads to other allergic diseases
(asthma, allergies)

Section 3
Symptoms of Psoriasis vs. Eczema

Symptoms of psoriasis and eczema go through a cycle: from being active (flare-ups) to a state of less active or inactive (remission) for a certain period of time, before the next flare-up gets triggered.

Similarities in symptoms

Both psoriasis and eczema share these common signs :

- Red patches or rashes (might appear purple in darker skin tone)
- Inflammation
- Skin dryness
- Itchiness
- Non-contagious, but are at higher risk of infections.
- Can appear anywhere on the body

- May cause skin cracks and bleeding due to friction or constant scratching

Due to these similar symptoms, you might get confused and misdiagnose either of the conditions, especially in infants and children. Hence, it is crucial to consult your doctor, specifically a trained dermatologist who can distinguish between the two skin conditions.

Differentiating Psoriasis From Eczema

Some differences may seem to overlap, but there are typical symptoms more evident in psoriasis than the other and vice versa.

PSORIASIS	ECZEMA
More inflamed, can be painful or sting.	Less inflamed than psoriasis.
Mild to moderate dryness and itchiness.	Extremely dry and intense itchiness due to weak skin barrier.

Appears thicker and raised from the skin like an extra layer.	Appears thinner but can be swollen.
Usually covered in rough white or silver scales (plaques) due to the buildup of dead skin cells.	Sometimes, the patches ooze fluids when there is an infection.
The borders surrounding the flares are clearer and more obvious.	Borders are less sharp and not as clear.
Usually found on the open areas: front of knees, outer elbows, the scalp, lower back, buttocks, and fingernails or toenails.	Often found on opposite areas of psoriasis where the skin folds: back of knees, inner elbows, the neck, ankles, wrists, hands, and possibly the face area.
Commonly associated with joint pains (psoriatic arthritis, diabetes, and cardiovascular diseases.	Commonly associated with diseases caused by allergies such as hay fever and asthma.

Can I Have Both Eczema and Psoriasis?

It is quite uncommon to have psoriasis and eczema at the same time. So far, not much research has been done to determine if psoriasis and eczema can coexist. Only 5 out of 354 children were found to have both psoriasis and eczema concurrently in one study; however, adults were not included in the study's sample.

However, you can suffer from eczema as a youngster, which would eventually go away, and then you might grow up to get psoriasis.

Section 4
Diagnosis of Psoriasis and Eczema

Dermatologists are the professionals best qualified to diagnose skin diseases. With just a physical examination, they can typically diagnose psoriasis or eczema. If more information is needed, skin examinations including skin biopsies and patch testing may be carried out.

Physical Examination

You might be questioned about your current symptoms throughout the procedure, and they might include things like:

- Where do the symptoms appear on your body?
- When did you start having them?
- How frequent are the flare-ups?
- Were you in contact with any harsh substances?
- Do you have existing allergies?

- How intense are the symptoms from mild, to moderate to severe?
- Did you experience any stress?
- Do any of your family members have a history of eczema or psoriasis?

If you use any cosmetic products or hygiene items that include irritating components, your dermatologist might also want to know about them.

It's a good idea to share as much information as you can to help receive an accurate diagnosis of your symptoms, since psoriasis can easily be confused for eczema. Do not self-diagnose or take over-the-counter medications without first visiting a clinician.

Skin Patch Test

In order to perform this painless test, many skin patches containing various substances (allergens) are applied, commonly taped to your back for two days. You are not permitted to get them wet during this time, so avoid exercising and take great care when taking a shower.

Before making a diagnosis, your dermatologist will monitor any reactions to the allergens for up to four days after they have been removed.

Since eczema and allergies are closely related, this test is usually used to diagnose eczema.

Skin Biopsy

Skin biopsy is a useful method for identifying eczema and for diagnosing skin disorders that go below the surface, such as psoriasis. It's a quick operation that takes place in your doctor's office to take a sample of skin tissue.

Also referred to as a punch biopsy, the procedure involves puncturing the skin as deeply as 2 to 3 mm with a tiny tube-like device in order to remove all three layers of skin. After that, the skin sample is brought to the lab for additional microscopic examination.

In order to numb the area and reduce or eliminate discomfort, anesthesia is given first; nonetheless, soreness is anticipated subsequently. It could take three weeks or perhaps a month for the biopsy wound to heal.

Section 5

Psoriasis & Eczema Triggers

In addition to having several symptoms in common, psoriasis and eczema also have some triggers.

Similarities in Triggers

Prolonged exposure to sunshine or excessively low temperatures can exacerbate itching, which is what causes both types of weather. Furthermore, experiencing frequent or high levels of emotional stress may lower cortisol levels, which are helpful in reducing inflammation and infection. This weakens the immune system and may be the reason why flare-ups occur.

An increased inflammatory response can result from psoriasis's overabundance of immune cells, eczema's extremely sensitive immune system, skin infections, and skin traumas. Cuts, scrapes, burns, and injections are examples of skin traumas.

Other Psoriasis Triggers

Additional factors that can cause psoriasis include drug use that interferes with the immune system's natural function, such as:

- **Drinking alcohol and smoking:** These substances might overstimulate your immune system and cause it to become hyperactive.

- **Some common pharmaceuticals:** These include blood pressure medications, antimalarials for malaria, and lithium for bipolar illness.

Other Eczema Triggers

The majority of external substances that might irritate the skin and cause eczema include:

- Personal hygiene and cosmetic items: shampoo, soap, body wash, and makeup

- Chemicals found in the home: dish soap, fabric and floor detergents, disinfectants

- Products with scents: essential oils, perfumes, scents, and scented goods
- Allergen exposure: dust, pollen, pet fur, smoke from cigarettes or fires, specific fabrics, and food
- Jewelry

Excessive perspiration can also be a problem for someone with eczema, particularly in high-sweat areas like the neck, inner elbow, and back of the knees. Sweats are known to cause irritation because they include sodium, or salt, which increases body heat and moisture loss.

Section 6

Treatments for Psoriasis and Eczema

While there are no known treatments for chronic, long-term diseases like eczema and psoriasis, physicians advise treating symptoms instead of the cause. Medication, phototherapy, herbal medicines, and self-care practices are common forms of treatment.

Based on the type of psoriasis or eczema, the severity of symptoms, and the potential for side effects, dermatologists propose treatment strategies.

Topical medications

Since topical treatments can be applied directly to the skin to alleviate inflammation and itching, they are the most critical item for anyone with psoriasis or eczema.

The following is a list of topical drugs:

- **Corticosteroids:** found in a variety of formulations, including sprays, ointments, gels, creams, and lotions. can, in extreme circumstances, also be taken orally.

- **Ceramides:** By fortifying the compromised skin barriers, this miracle product for dry skin helps seal in moisture and promote skin restoration. Ceramides are an ingredient in several moisturizers for skin care.

- **Salicylic acid (SA):** Attempts to soften and thin the psoriasis plaques. A larger dose, however, may make your inflammation worse. The recommended range is 2% to 10%.

- **Emollients:** Used as a moisturizer to moisten the skin and reduce irritation.

Phototherapy

When topical treatments fail to alleviate a person's severe psoriasis or eczema, phototherapy—also known as light therapy—is utilized. Additionally, it can serve as an effective treatment for symptoms that affect a broad portion of the body.

Because this procedure uses a specialized machine that produces UV radiation, which helps to slow down cell growth and reduce inflammation, it should only be used by a dermatologist or healthcare expert.

Phototherapy is not a one-time treatment; it normally takes numerous medical visits, up to two months, and is tapered off gradually as the symptoms improve. It's crucial to discuss the potential adverse effects of phototherapy with your physician.

Oral or Injected Medications

For those with moderate to severe symptoms, oral drugs (in the form of pills or liquids) and injectable shots may be a better option than topical therapies and light therapy alone.

Healthcare professionals usually suggest short-term use or modest use in conjunction with topical treatments due to potential side effects.

To prevent drug abuse, you should need a prescription for these medications from your doctor:

- **Antihistamines:** Aids in itching relief.

- **Antibiotics:** Best used for infections that might be brought on by persistent scratching.

- **Systemic drugs or immunosuppressants:** Cyclosporine and methotrexate work on the entire immune system to suppress hyperactive reactions and lessen flare-ups. But because these medications have a lot of adverse effects, they should only be taken as needed.

- **Vitamin D synthetics or analogues:** Renowned to lower overall inflammation and strengthen the skin barrier in eczema sufferers. Tacalcitol, calcitriol, and calcipotriol are a few examples.

- **Biologics:** Has a similar effect to immunosuppressants in that it lessens the intensity of symptoms. Typically administered by injections or intravenous (IV) infusions into the bloodstream.

Do note that not all forms of treatment are suitable for everyone. Discuss with your doctor about the potential side effects and your suitability for each treatment option.

Natural Remedies for Psoriasis And Eczema

Since Psoriasis and eczema are chronic, the goal is usually not to cure them, but to control their symptoms and prevent flare-ups. Here are 19 natural remedies you can try at home to manage symptoms psoriasis and eczema:

Aloe Vera Gel

Given that aloe vera is moisturizing, antioxidant, antimicrobial, immune-boosting and wound-healing, it is no wonder that aloe vera gel can alleviate the symptoms of Psoriasis and eczema.

Applying aloe vera gel after cleaning the affected skin with unscented soap and water can help to moisturize dry skin, minimize the risk of skin infection, and aid the healing of broken skin.

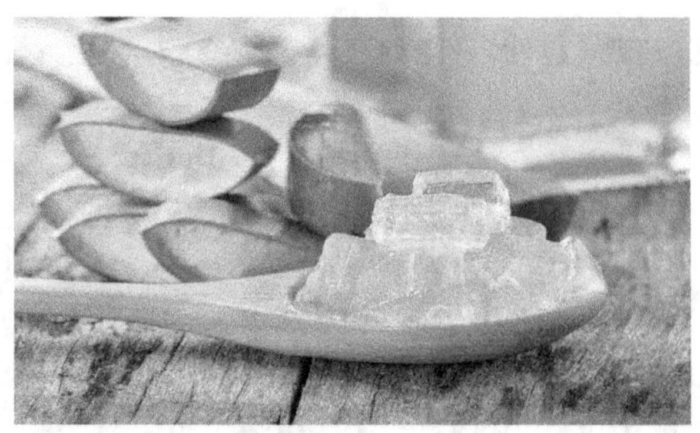

Apple Cider Vinegar

Soaps, shampoos, cosmetics and even tap water can affect your skin's pH levels, which is why soap is a common Psoriasis and eczema trigger. Apple cider vinegar, a mild acid, may help to restore your skin's pH levels.

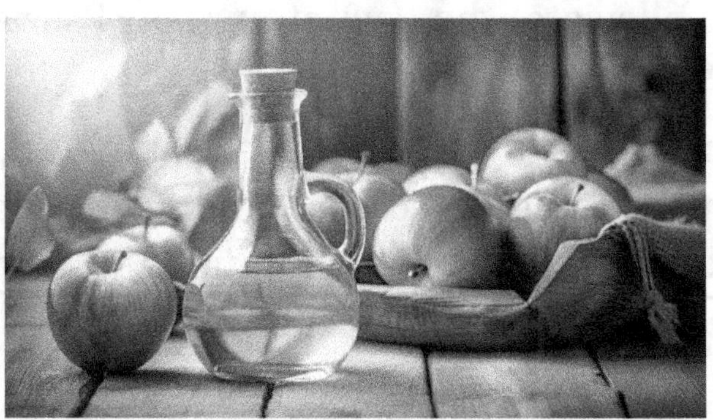

A simple way to use apple cider vinegar to treat Psoriasis and eczema is to add it to your lukewarm bath water, soak in it for 15 to 20 minutes, then rinse off with cool water. You can also create a moisturizer, facial toner, hair oil, and wet wrap containing apple cider vinegar.

Cool Compress

The itching that comes with Psoriasis and eczema can be unbearable, but scratching does more harm than good and damages your skin further.

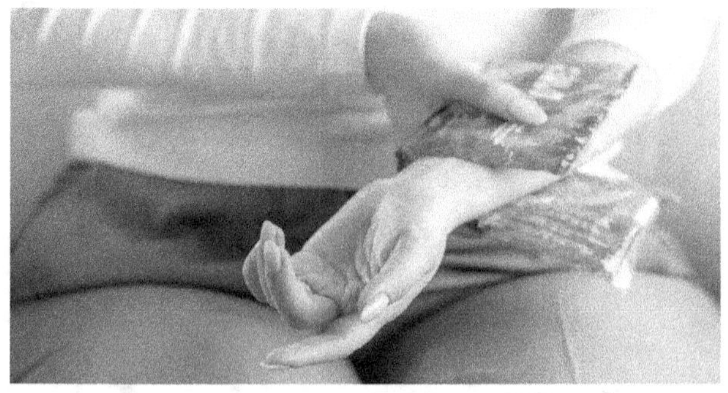

Applying a cool compress by placing a clean damp cloth on the affected area of skin can ease itching.

Lukewarm showers & baths

Frequent, hot baths and showers can dry out your skin, triggering a Psoriasis and Eczema flare-up. Take short, lukewarm showers or baths instead, and pat yourself dry gently instead of rubbing hard. Remember to also apply moisturizer afterwards.

Bleach

A small amount of bleach mixed into bath water can kill the infection-causing bacteria on our skin, easing inflammation, itching, and scaling. To create a bleach bath, simply add half a cup of household bleach into a full tub of water. Soak in it for 10 minutes, then rinse off with cool water.

Take note that chlorine may be problematic for some people, so it is best to consult with your doctor before trying this remedy and/or test it out on a small area of skin first.

Colloidal Oatmeal

Colloidal oatmeal, or *Avena sativa*, refers to finely ground oat grains known to have skin-healing properties. You can add it to your bath and soak in it, or apply it as a paste on your skin.

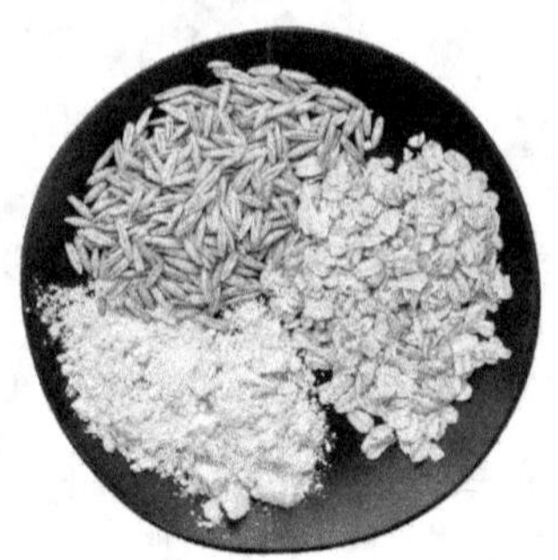

While colloidal oatmeal is safe to use for most people, those with an allergy to oats should avoid it. Manufacturers often process oats with wheat, so those with a gluten allergy should take extra precaution as well. Alternatively, you can try baking soda in place of colloidal oatmeal.

Coconut oil

Besides the moisturizing properties of the fatty acids it contains, virgin coconut oil may help to combat infections and inflammation. You can apply coconut oil to your skin directly several times a day, especially after a bath or shower and before bed.

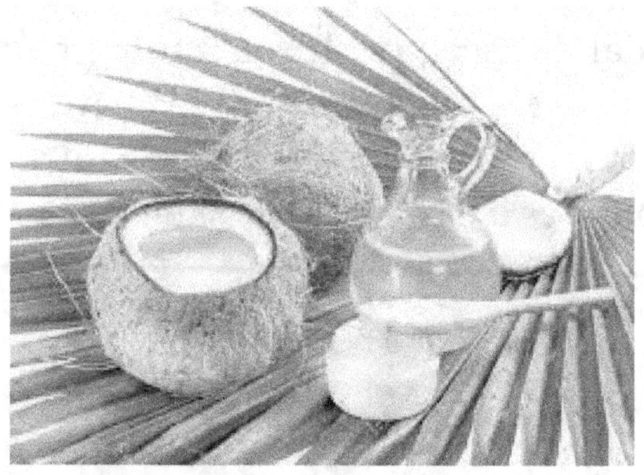

Make sure to only use cold-pressed virgin coconut oil for your skin. Those who are allergic to coconuts should also avoid this remedy.

Honey

With its anti-inflammatory, antioxidant, and antimicrobial properties, honey may be able to ease and reduce the symptoms of Psoriasis and Eczema. To use honey for Psoriasis and Eczema lesions, apply a thin layer of medical-grade honey to the affected area and cover it with a gauze or bandage overnight. Gently remove the dressing and clean the area in the morning.

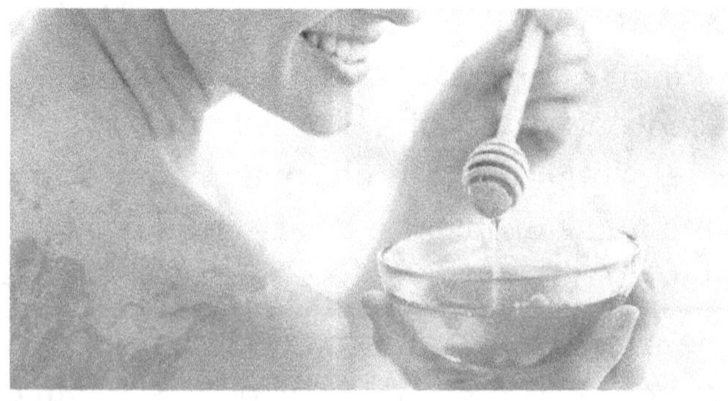

If it is your first time trying this remedy, make sure to do a patch test first to ensure you are not allergic to honey.

Tea Tree Oil

There are many potential benefits of using tea tree oil for treating Psoriasis and Eczema, including reducing inflammation, healing wounds, fighting bacteria and viruses, and relieving itch.

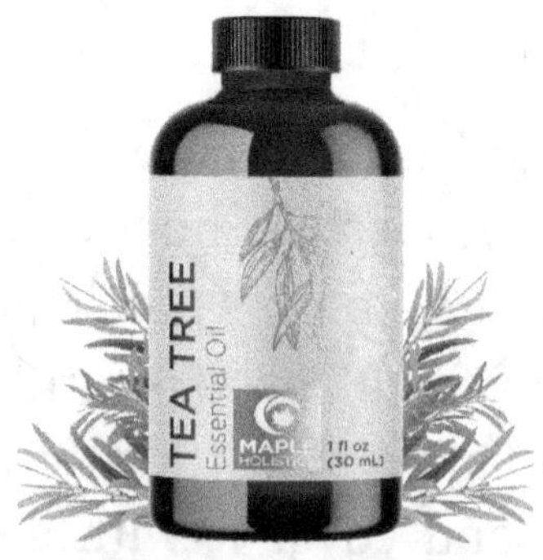

While it is generally safe to use tea tree oil on any external area of your body, make sure to use them safely as high concentrations can have adverse results instead. Most tea tree oil products are sold in low concentrations of 5% or less, but if you are using pure essential tea tree oil, make sure to dilute it by mixing a few drops into a carrier oil such as coconut or almond oil.

To be safe, always do a patch test first. You should also check with your doctor before applying tea tree oil to your skin to ensure it does not interfere with any ongoing forms of Psoriasis and Eczema treatment.

Diet

Some foods can cause inflammation, while others fight it. As Psoriasis and Eczema are conditions linked to inflammation, some people find that eating certain foods worsens or improves their Psoriasis and Eczema symptoms.

Reducing your intake of inflammatory food and adopting a diet rich in foods that fight inflammation can help soothe Psoriasis and Eczema symptoms. An anti-inflammatory diet includes food like:

- Fatty fish, such as salmon, mackerel and sardines
- Fruits, such as strawberries, blueberries, and oranges
- Leafy greens, such as spinach and kale
- Olive oil
- Nuts, such as almonds and walnuts
- Tomatoes

Soaps

Harsh soaps can irritate our skin and worsen symptoms of Psoriasis and Eczema. Our skin's natural pH is 4 to 5, while the pH of soap is 9 to 10, which can result in a pH imbalance and dry out our skin.

Here are some tips when showering: Choose a mild soap that is superfatted, non alkaline, and free of sodium lauryl sulfate and exfoliating. Make sure to rinse off completely to avoid any soap residue after bathing. Be gentle on the skin when showering or bathing and do not use a washcloth, sponge, loofah, or scrub that might scrape your skin and irritate it further. Dry off gently by patting rather than rubbing, and moisturize immediately to seal in moisture.

Detergent and Softener

Laundry detergent tends to contain harsh chemicals, such as lathering agents, that can dry out the skin and worsen Psoriasis and Eczema. Fabric softeners also often result in fragrances and other chemicals lingering on clothes, irritating your skin.

If you suspect that this might be an issue, try switching your detergent to one that is milder, fragrance-free or color-free, and skip the fabric softener altogether.

Avoid Extreme Temperatures

Hot temperatures can trigger the prickly, itchy feeling on our skin and cause perspiration, which may encourage the growth of bacteria and other skin irritants. Meanwhile, cold winters tend to have dry air, resulting in dry skin which can worsen Psoriasis and Eczema symptoms.

During hot weather, wear loose and breathable clothing, stay hydrated, bring soft paper wipes to stay dry, and stay in the cool indoors as much as possible, especially during the hottest hours of the day. During cold and dry winters, use a humidifier, wear the appropriate gears (take note to avoid using materials that may irritate your skin, such as wool), and moisturize frequently.

If severe eczema is causing major inconveniences and affecting your day-to-day life, an extreme measure will be to move to a place with a different climate.

Moisturise

Moisturising has been mentioned multiple times in this study, but it cannot be stressed enough. Besides the frequency of moisturizing, using the right moisturizer is key. Avoid lotions that contain fragrances and other potential irritants.

Sunflower oil

Virgin sunflower seed oil can help your skin retain moisture and has anti-inflammatory properties that may alleviate the symptoms of eczema. Simply apply it onto your skin twice a day. However, avoid this remedy if you are allergic to sunflower seeds.

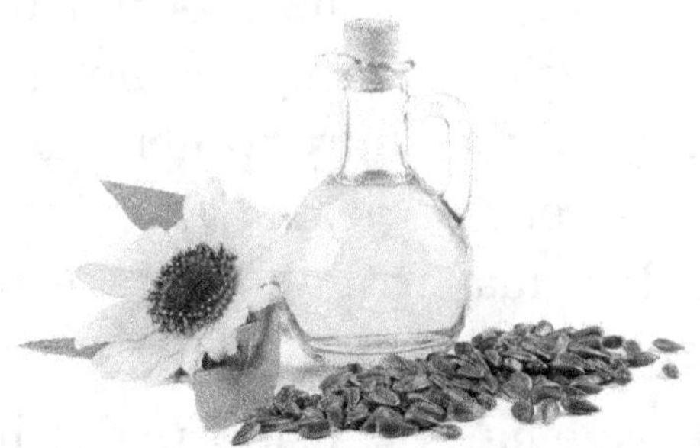

Acupressure

Preliminary findings from a study conducted by Northwestern University have revealed that pressing on a specific point on your arm may help to reduce itching caused by Psoriasis and Eczema. To find this acupressure point, place your right hand over your left elbow while your left arm is bent, then feel for the top of the forearm muscle. Massage this spot for 3 minutes while taking deep breaths.

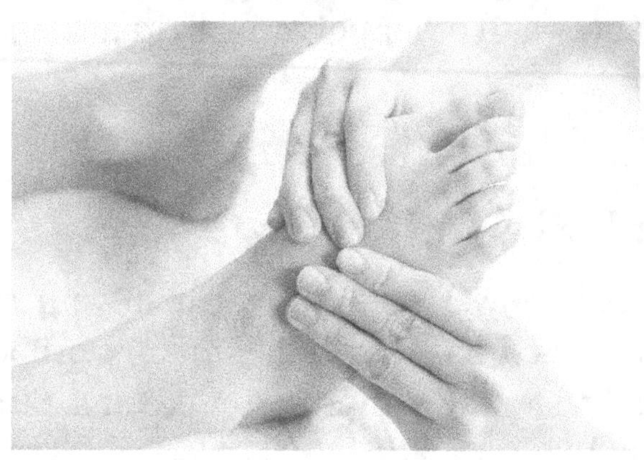

While more in-depth and large-scale studies are required to confirm these findings, the initial findings are promising and there's no harm trying it out.

Avoid High-Intensity Exercises

During an eczema flare-up, body heat and perspiration can worsen the itch and symptoms. While it is still important to exercise to stay healthy, there are some measures you can take to reduce the aggravation:

- Work out in an air-conditioned area indoors or when the temperature is cooler outdoors
- Hydrate adequately
- Take frequent breaks to let your body cool down
- Keep a towel close to wipe off sweat as you work out
- Wearing light, breathable and loose cotton clothing
- Shower shortly after your exercise session

Avoid scratching

Itchiness is one of the hardest Psoriasis and Eczema symptoms to deal with, and telling you to avoid scratching is much easier said than done. However, scratching can trigger the release of inflammatory substances and worsen the itch. It can also lead to broken skin, increasing the chances of an infection.

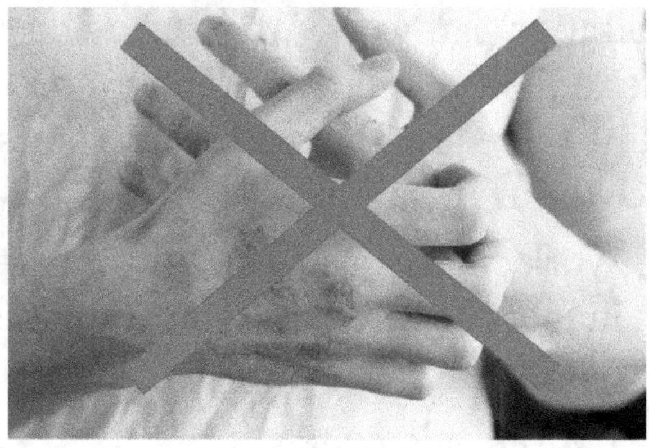

To minimize the damage from scratching, always keep your nails trimmed. You may also want to wrap up the affected area and wear gloves to sleep.

De-stress

Stress, which often leads to inflammation in the body, is a common eczema trigger. If you find yourself under stress, try some relaxation techniques such as meditation, deep breathing and yoga. Different techniques work for different individuals, so find something that works for you.

A generally healthy lifestyle of having a balanced diet, getting plenty of sleep, and regular exercise, can also help to reduce the chances of a Psoriasis and Eczema flare-up.

Remember: Whenever you are trying out new products and remedies, always test a modest amount on a small area of skin first, in case of allergy or irritation. If in doubt, always consult your doctor.

Self-care Precautions

Apart from medications and therapy, you can make small changes to your daily habits by being extra careful :

- Ensure the water is set to lukewarm during showers and the sessions short.

- Avoid rubbing or wiping your body harshly after showers. Instead, pat your skin gently and let the air dry it naturally.

- Apply moisturizers daily and immediately after showers (while your skin is still damp). Opt for oil-based moisturizers such as body butter,

- Wear loose clothes and non-abrasive fabrics including towels.

- Use a humidifier, especially at night when the temperature is cold and dry. Humidifiers increase the moisture level in the air which can relieve your dry skin. Be careful not to adjust the humidity too high, as damp air may result in the growth of bacteria.

- Choose hygiene, skincare, and cosmetics products that contain gentle ingredients or those specially formulated for psoriasis and eczema. Steer clear of those that are unsuitable for skin dryness such as foam cleansers and water-based moisturizers.

- Avoid being under the sun and in an air-conditioned room for too long.

- Minimize participating in rigorous activities like intense workouts that can lead to excessive sweating and increased body heat.

- Include anti-inflammatory foods in your diet for example fishes rich in omega-3 fatty acids, ginger, nuts, leafy vegetables, and antioxidant-rich fruits.

- Keep your fingernails and toenails short to avoid bleeding in care

- Be extra alert of the triggers.

Section 7

Prevention is better than cure

Finding the triggers and preventing psoriasis and eczema flare-ups altogether is a better long-term strategy for managing eczema symptoms, even though home remedies and treatments can assist.

Make a note of everything you eat and anything else that irritates you. You can even keep track of eczema flare-ups and record exposure to possible causes by keeping a journal, if that helps. After you've determined what triggers them, take action to keep them from ever leading to an exacerbation of your eczema. For instance, if sweating is a trigger for you, always keep moisturizing tissues on hand and take a shower soon after working out.

Eczema and psoriasis can be difficult to manage, but with perseverance, self-control, and the correct assistance, you can learn more about your body and avoid flare-ups of eczema. When in doubt, consult a physician to create a strategy that suits your needs.